Cambridge Elements ≡

Elements in Emergency Neurosurgery
edited by
Nihal Gurusinghe
Lancashire Teaching Hospital NHS Trust
Peter Hutchinson
University of Cambridge, Society of British Neurological Surgeons and Royal College of Surgeons of England
Ioannis Fouyas
Royal College of Surgeons of Edinbur
Naomi Slator
North Bristol NHS Trust
Ian Kamaly-Asl
Royal Manchester Children's Hospit
Peter Whitfield
University Hospitals Plymouth NHS Trust

T0334115

NEUROSURGICAL HANDOVERS AND STANDARDS FOR EMERGENCY CARE

Simon Lammy
Institute of Neurological Sciences
Jennifer Brown
Institute of Neurological Sciences

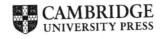

CAMBRIDGE
UNIVERSITY PRESS

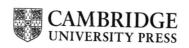

Shaftesbury Road, Cambridge CB2 8EA, United Kingdom

One Liberty Plaza, 20th Floor, New York, NY 10006, USA

477 Williamstown Road, Port Melbourne, VIC 3207, Australia

314–321, 3rd Floor, Plot 3, Splendor Forum, Jasola District Centre,
New Delhi – 110025, India

103 Penang Road, #05–06/07, Visioncrest Commercial, Singapore 238467

Cambridge University Press is part of Cambridge University Press & Assessment,
a department of the University of Cambridge.

We share the University's mission to contribute to society through the pursuit of
education, learning and research at the highest international levels of excellence.

www.cambridge.org
Information on this title: www.cambridge.org/9781009548458

DOI: 10.1017/9781009548502

First published 2024

A catalogue record for this publication is available from the British Library

ISBN 978-1-009-54845-8 Paperback
ISSN 2755-0656 (online)
ISSN 2755-0648 (print)

Cambridge University Press & Assessment has no responsibility for the persistence or
accuracy of URLs for external or third-party internet websites referred to in this
publication and does not guarantee that any content on such websites is, or will
remain, accurate or appropriate.

Every effort has been made in preparing this Element to provide accurate and
up-to-date information which is in accord with accepted standards and practice at the
time of publication. Although case histories are drawn from actual cases, every effort
has been made to disguise the identities of the individuals involved. Nevertheless, the
authors, editors and publishers can make no warranties that the information
contained herein is totally free from error, not least because clinical standards are
constantly changing through research and regulation. The authors, editors and
publishers therefore disclaim all liability for direct or consequential damages resulting
from the use of material contained in this Element. Readers are strongly advised to pay
careful attention to information provided by the manufacturer of any drugs or
equipment that they plan to use.

Neurosurgical Handovers and Standards for Emergency Care

Elements in Emergency Neurosurgery

DOI: 10.1017/9781009548502
First published online: December 2024

Simon Lammy
Institute of Neurological Sciences

Jennifer Brown
Institute of Neurological Sciences

Author for correspondence: Simon Lammy, simon.lammy@glasgow.ac.uk

Abstract: One of the biggest challenges as a neurosurgical trainee is to master the handover. This requires developing an organisational efficiency to concisely relay relevant patient information to a suitably qualified person to execute a given task. A trainee can work extremely hard during an on-call, making suitable decisions, implementing previous plans to perfection and covering slack in a team. But if the presentation of this work is unclear then it undoes a lot of that hard work and generates an impression of a trainee being disorganised. Success in a handover requires an understanding of whom you are talking to, what you are saying, how you are saying it and if the way you are communicating gains and maintains interest. Above all a handover should ensure the smooth continuity of care of a patient.

Keywords: handover, organisation, efficiency, robust, honesty

ISBNs: 9781009548458 (PB), 9781009548502 (OC)
ISSNs: 2755-0656 (online), 2755-0648 (print)

Contents

It is 7 a.m. and you are coming to the end of your twenty-four-hour resident on-call. You are operating on a trauma patient, evacuating an acute subdural haematoma. You are aware that a thirteen-year-old is coming to paediatric ITU intubated with a subarachnoid haemorrhage, a thirty-five-year-old woman is deteriorating upstairs from mass effect from a very large right temporal glioblastoma and this current on table case has required a major haemorrhage protocol. You wish to quickly finish to attend to these patients, go round ITU and HDU, and check on the patient going to CT to exclude a re-haemorrhage from an AVM, and any other critical care-related issues to enable you to prepare for handover at 8.30 a.m. But the computer system is down and your on-call spreadsheet is inaccessible. To make things worse, you forgot to message your SpR colleagues so someone can come in early to relieve you in the theatre. Help!

Introduction

The quick and rapidly changing nature of a neurosurgical on-call means trainees need to develop and then maintain a high degree of alertness to ensure the understanding, documentation and discussion of each patient's information and plans are as robust as possible and understood by everyone involved in the patient's ongoing care. For example, what is the plan if the motor score drops in a patient being monitored with post-haemorrhagic hydrocephalus? Repeat CT? Go straight to EVD? LP? Or is the consultant's preference if the aqueduct is unobstructed to have a lumbar drain inserted as it is quicker and avoids a general anaesthetic? These questions apply to inpatients housed in a neurosurgical building as well as those in referring hospitals.

This example above is relatively straightforward but all too commonly dubiety exists especially after a change of shifts. If you factor in consultants' individual preferences based on a combination of their own experience and clinical factors affecting the decision for that specific patient, then the decision-making of the neurosurgical SpR can become very complex and nuanced. A neurosurgical handover must ensure consultant preferences are highlighted. There is a particular onus on senior registrars to help junior colleagues navigate these nuances, but there is an onus on all trainees to keep the consultant informed and to understand and document plans.

Diagnostic and management dilemmas are not unique to neurosurgery. Robust handover arrangements are an expected professional standard across all medical and surgical specialties and are laid out in Good Medical Practice, Domain 3: Colleagues, Culture and Safety as published by the General Medical Council (GMC) the governing and licensing body of doctors in the United Kingdom.[1] This emphasises the importance of individual clinicians contributing to the safe transfer of patients and their information between various healthcare professionals and trusts (see Text Box 1).

Box 1 Good Medical Practice

1. 'Promptly share all relevant information about patients (including any reasonable adjustments and communication support preferences) with others involved in their care, within and across teams, as required'.
2. 'Share information with patients about the progress of their care, who is responsible for which aspect of their care, the name of the lead clinician or team with overall responsibility for their care'.
3. 'Be confident that information necessary for ongoing care has been shared before you go off duty, before you delegate care, or before you refer the patient to another health or social care provider'.
4. 'Check, where practical, that a named clinician or team has taken over responsibility when your role in a patient's care has ended'.

Furthermore, an expectation of neurosurgical SpRs is to be certain that the delegation of ongoing care of a patient should ideally go to a colleague who has the necessary skills and experience to manage that patient, for example a head-injured patient coming directly to theatre for evacuation of a haemorrhage overlying a sinus needs a trainee to quickly recognise the potential challenges of such a case and are expected to involve the consultant in decision-making, and perhaps direct involvement surgically, due to the seriousness of the situation. This is a classic example of a case demanding consultant input irrespective of the trainees' experience.

The purpose of this section is to summarise the salient points of neurosurgical handover and documentation to enable efficient continuity of care of inpatients and ward attenders. It shall employ a direct and concise approach.

Definition

The purpose of a handover is to ensure uninterrupted forward momentum to a patient's care employing designated individuals of appropriate competency and experience to execute a task. It is a two-way exchange of information to create an awareness of pressing clinical issues about patients under a team's care, pertinent information about patients about to come under that team's care, accurate transfer of information about prioritised tasks and management plans, and a knowledge of potential anticipated changes to such plans if the clinical need dictates a change.[2]

Therefore, a merely *good* handover ensures ongoing care which does not compromise patient safety,[3] for example SpR A 'this patient arrived three hours ago and needs a left-sided L4/5 microdiscectomy for incomplete cauda equina syndrome tonight'. However, an _excellent_ handover enables a new team to enact a previously devised plan with minimal interruption, for example SpR B 'this patient arrived three hours ago and needs a left-sided L4/5 microdiscectomy for incomplete cauda equina syndrome, is consented and marked (but please double check these), the image intensifier has been requested, the radiographer is aware, the anaesthetist has already seen the patient and their admission documented in their case notes'. We should aspire to _excellence_ not merely being _good_ at work.

An excellent handover reflects an organisational efficiency which anticipates challenges and pre-emptively provides solutions for the incoming team. There are simple ways to optimise a handover and these should be continually reviewed as part of the audit pillar of clinical govrnance.[4]

Structure of Handover

The success of a neurosurgical handover depends on some core ingredients (see Text Box 2). These include mandating relevant individuals to be present, strong leadership through an accepted model of which clinician is in charge of coordinating proceedings, a designated time for handover which has been agreed upon at a departmental level and a structure to proceedings which prioritises patients according to an accepted model of how the service is run. Fundamentally, for this to work all attendees should embrace punctuality and come prepared to receive, give, understand and question information being discussed so that the very best in patient care can be delivered based on local and regional expertise. The morning handover in neurosurgery is a core component of service delivery. It is a workhorse in which decisions are made and invaluable learning occurs if trainees take note of divergences of opinion at the consultant level which reflect the nuances of neurosurgical practice.

BOX 2 CORE INGREDIENTS

1. Core attendees
2. Strong leadership
3. Time
4. Structure
5. Punctuality
6. Preparedness

Time

Having a time rendered sacrosanct across a department and an expectation for participation optimises attendance and elevates the standard of decision-making through robust discussion. This time should coincide with the on-call team finishing and a subsequent on-call team beginning and ultimately these should be harmonised, for example in Glasgow all three tiers of neurosurgeon: consultants, registrars and senior house officers participate in a unified post-on-call registrar led handover which begins at 8.30 a.m. Therefore, a call to attention at the appointed time does not surprise anyone and should be an expected fulcrum on which the working day is hinged. Being punctual should be considered a professional expectation (not a courtesy).

Location

Once a dedicated time has been allocated, a location to conduct proceedings conducive to a robust discussion of business needs to be found. This should be a room which permits easy visualisation of scans, for example has a large projector screen, and quiet surroundings to enable clear communication of business. This room should not be open to interruption and disturbance from colleagues. In Glasgow, prior to the COVID pandemic, the handover was conducted in a radiology room having rows for each grade of surgeon. This has been replaced by an MS Teams-based meeting.

Attendance

A departmental handover requires attendance by consultants, registrars, senior house officers and clinical nurse specialists. The usual core individuals include the outgoing on-call registrar and consultant, incoming on-call registrar and consultant and a registrar representative for each of the relevant teams and specialities in case issues for those teams and specialities patients' have come up. Local departmental structure and practice will determine the individuals required to attend each day.

Leadership

The post-on-call registrar usually runs a departmental handover but the post-on-call consultant is responsible for ensuring it runs according to established departmental practice. These distinct but subtle differences, if clearly defined, enable the person most knowledgeable of intricate patient details (registrar) to have space to run proceedings, and the person having overall responsibility for the on-call (consultant) to ensure unnecessary interruption and excessive discussion are kept to a minimum.

Ultimately, being a registrar in charge of handover requires staying focused, handing over salient points in a patient's presentation, preventing degeneracy into excessive discussion and to reconfirm plans.[5]

Organisation

Employing a tried and tested format which is known through the department is crucial to organising one's thoughts and is important for an excellent handover. Preparing for handover by being in the room beforehand to preload scans consciously highlights to an exhausted mind blind spots in one's presentational organisation and if one's individual decision-making is robust enough to weather scrutiny if questioned. Having a handover document detailing the order is crucial.

Delivery

A quick introduction to bring everyone to awareness that handover is beginning should be done. A clear and concise diction is important and sets the tone for a quick and efficient handover. An example of a tried and tested format is to begin detailing overnight operations, emergency admissions, expected admissions and team and speciality referrals. This style is unique to our unit in Glasgow. Therefore, a deviation from it in Glasgow would be unexpected and not encouraged. So understanding one's local neurosurgical unit's style is paramount to success in that unit and variations do exist (see Text Box 3).

Communication should be clear. A common misconception is to be quiet out of a sense of humility. Although one should not be over-confident a degree of confidence and clarity in diction is important to gain and maintain attention. We caution being in haste as this does not permit colleagues to understand plans.

Box 3 Handover Presentation Order

Emergency Operations
Emergency Admissions
Expected Admissions
Specialty Specific
    Paediatrics
    Vascular
    Oncology
    Spine
    Functional
    General

Clear summary statements are more valuable when communicating than rapid speech that includes every detail. Some referrals are hard work, or even quite frustrating, and require the referrer to gather more information and call again. There may be inaccuracies and misconceptions to work through. A detailed account of this process is seldom relevant or valuable to the incoming team. Handover requires practice and experience. If colleagues are unsure of what you have said simply slow it down and repeat it. If scans need to be shown to support the presentation, try to select relevant sequences and cuts in advance. Display an informative image, or set of images, and avoid constant fidgeting with the controls. This leaves the audience wondering what you are trying to show.

Style

Adhere to a presentation style which is congruent to the department's usual manner, for example in Glasgow our style is name, age, referring hospital, diagnosis, relevant previous medical history, and presenting complaint, examination findings, management plan advised and plan for subsequent on-call teams to be aware of, for example 'John Smith is a 65-year-old man currently in Wishaw who is on Apixaban for AF and has a moderate left-sided acute subdural haematoma. He had an intoxicated fall down fourteen stairs and is neurologically intact. We advised stopping his Apixaban and admitting him locally and repeating the CT in seven days to guide future management of the clot'. Some neurosurgical centres have a preference to present cases in a teaching style so consultants can question trainees. Irrespective of your centre's chosen style a simple dictum is to know the style and not deviate from it.

Communication

A core aspect of handover extends beyond discussing a case and debating a proposed management plan. Ensuring a named individual of appropriate experience and competency follows through on a plan is important, for example 'can a registrar on Miss Brown's team call Wishaw to inform them to do an MRI on this patient to look for blood breakdown products, please? Thank you, Nathan'. 'Can a neuro-oncology MDT form be submitted by a registrar on Mr. Hassan's team, please? Thank you, Mustafa'. If no registrar is present for a specific team then emailing that team's registrars is a way to communicate a plan. The importance of being clear delegating a task and requesting confirmation of acceptance cannot be underestimated. It is a GMC requirement for handover. It can be useful to check a colleague is listening by reaffirming a question or management plan, for example 'Miss Brown, is it OK for this patient to be discharged home?'. "Elsie, are you still happy to submit that MDT form?'

Ownership

Every patient should be the responsibility of a specific consultant. This individual should be named early in the discussion so that expectations for current inpatient and ongoing outpatient care is known to enable a patient to be managed accordingly.

Documentation

Each neurosurgical centre should have an electronic method to document referrals (see Grundy, Ioannides and Ray, *Sources, Modes and Triage of Emergency Referrals to Neurosurgery*, Elements in Emergency Neurosurgery, Cambridge University Press, forthcoming). This can include an MS Excel sheet but more commonly an electronic referral system which captures the exact wording of the referring team. The downside of the former is that there is potential for inaccuracies in understanding and documentation. This can give rise to clinical or more rarely, medicolegal difficulties.

An electronic system, for example such as Refer A Patient, enables real-time dialogue and documentation of what the referrer has said and what the on-call neurosurgical registrar has documented as a reply. These systems are recommended by countless Ombudsman reports. However, whatever system you use it is your duty to ensure it is up to date in real time, plans documented including names of consultants, dates and times of decisions and names of colleagues to enact these plans.

Overall

There should be no doubt in anyone's mind that a plan for each patient irrespective of their location has been made and understood by the relevant people in the room.

Documentation

It is a common misconception that handover only exists in a formal capacity in morning meetings or in an informal manner during night handovers between day and night teams, but it is an ongoing process. Documentation throughout all neurosurgical practice can serve as a means to highlight concerns, request things to be carried out and provide context to a patient situation that helps on-call teams quickly implement a plan if the clinical situation dictates an unexpected change to management. Three domains are common areas for mistakes or omissions to happen in the continuity of care of a patient: operation notes, inpatient ward round summaries and ward attenders. Remember, *if it is not documented it did not happen.*

Operation Notes

This is one of the most important documents in a patient's admission. If written well it enables an outside observer to have a clear insight into the indication for the operation, the technical aspects of the case, the findings and intended follow-up. However, a distinction between a merely _good_ operation note and an _excellent_ one should be made (see Text Box 4).

From experience making a detailed operation note has multiple benefits: (a) serves as an aide memoire for future cases, (b) acts as a future reference guide to an on-call team about a complex patients neurosurgical history if a repeat operation comes up in future, (c) is invaluable for other specialties involved in their care, (d) is usually the most accurate and concise place to document the indication for and preoperative neurological status of the patient and (e) can be extremely useful in court. One of the authors (Simon Lammy) has had occasions where he has been called to court only for the Crown to not require his attendance due to the detail of the operation note negating his presence.

We do not merely hand over to neurosurgeons, doctors and other healthcare professionals but to lawyers as well. Whatever we document can be scrutinised in a court of law. The RCS England has published generic guidelines on operation notes and these have been audited in Glasgow.[6]

Ward Rounds

Similarly, documentation from rounds although delegated to the junior most member of the team, for example FY1s and FY2s, does require accuracy of information and for this to have oversight by neurosurgical SpRs. The one place

---

Box 4 GOOD VERSUS EXCELLENT OPERATION NOTES

SpR A's Op Note 'Indication: blocked shunt and hydrocephalus on CT' gives a concise reason for the shunt to be explored but this is merely good if compared to

SpR B's Op Note 'Indication: worsening headache and visual obscuration. The CT demonstrates acute hydrocephalus. No CSF could be obtained from the proximal valve complex. This is consistent with the patients' 4× previous shunt revisions. These have included intraventricular haemorrhage due to choroid plexus adhesions to proximal catheter'.

The latter gives more detail in a concise manner which enables a neurosurgeon assessing and doing this patient's sixth shunt revision to be forewarned and therefore forearmed.

that causes agitation for on-call teams is if a delicate discussion with the patient's relatives has occurred but not been documented. Inconsistency, or repetition of important discussions such as DNA-CPR decisions, end of life care and drastic changes to expected management plans undermine the family's confidence in care and could cause significant family distress.

Above all nuances exist in patient management due to the quickly changing nature of how neural tissue behaves under critical conditions. Reasons for changes in plans such as cancelling planned surgery for a patient intended for VP shunt revision who improves due to a correction of metabolic disturbance, need to be documented. This will be especially valuable if they become confused again later or if they have persistent ventriculomegaly.

Ward Attenders and Urgent Outpatient Reviews

This category of patients can present specific challenges namely that of a decision and follow-up. Oftentimes the responsible consultant is not available to ask for a definitive decision on a ward attender, and this decision gets delayed. Remembering to document accurately the clinical assessment and set a reminder to discuss the case next time that consultant is around requires an organisational efficiency that can be more difficult than a hectic on-call. Why? Because unless the patient attending has a simple problem, and other consultants can step in to make a decision their colleague trusts, a trainee can spend several days chasing a decision.

The patient may present again during this interval. Furthermore, if detailed imaging is needed organising this for a future date can be difficult. A solution is to always know a ward attender's neurosurgical issue in detail and organise imaging in advance. A frustration of MRI radiographers is that several subacute presentations may be seen on the same day with each reviewing registrar expecting a 'same day' scan, for example, for worsening lumbar radiculopathy and some slight sphincter disturbance. It should be possible to organise most subacute reviews in advance to ease the often-hectic schedules of imaging departments.

Pitfalls

Systemic Issues

The need to multitask can present specific challenges. One registrar may be responsible to more than one on-call consultant if the unit has a split rota. If you are being pulled in too many ways, get help from a colleague or the consultant on-call. The registrar may be scrubbed when handover time arrives. This is more common as units trend toward shift systems with several handovers per day. In our department a twenty-four-hour single resident on-call was usual until recently.

In general, it was easy to find a colleague to take over a theatre case to free the on-call registrar to organise their handover at 8.30 a.m. A newer twelve-hour two-tier shift-based working pattern means that potential for failure exists particularly at evening handover when not many colleagues are arriving, just the oncoming on-call team. It is usually simplest in this circumstance for the incoming senior SpR to complete the case whilst the outgoing junior and senior SpRs handover to the incoming junior SpR.

Naturally, any system having more people involved increases the risk of things being forgotten, lost or misremembered by mistakenly thinking someone else is sorting it out. This can increase the tension at times of handing over. A suggestion is to always be aware of potential future happenings. If you anticipate being scrubbed during handover then alert your colleagues to come to the theatre, ensure the on-call database is as up to date as it can be and highlight things which need attention as much as you can.

Delegation and Multiple Responsibilities

Another potential pitfall is to assume that because the next step in a patient's care is clear, someone is taking charge of that task. It can be frustrating and embarrassing if a week or more passes before omissions such as organising scans, review of ward attenders, completion of operation notes, submission of MDT forms are recognised. Worse, patients may come to harm because of such delays.

So, agree a plan that includes 'who' as well as 'what' at handover. A simple rule of thumb for an operation is that if you have done it to take sole responsibility for the operation note, post-op scans (blaming the ward doctor for a post-MRI scan request not being submitted reflects badly on you especially as you know more about the nuances of a case to get it vetted and done), relevant MDT forms, other speciality discussions, discharge and follow up plans. The same goes for handover. If you know more about a case it simply makes sense for you to action things. This ensures smoother and faster communication and completion of tasks.

But, due to the ever-growing complexity of neurosurgical practice, time is not a renewable resource. So if one is stretched, one should endeavour to ask for help from a colleague who is competent to execute the task.

Conclusions

Covering an acute speciality on-call can be very rewarding as there is potential for preventing rapid deterioration and sometimes dramatic or unexpected recovery. It can also include a significant burden of repetitive or mundane work. The exciting and the mundane alike need clear documentation and sound handover. Documenting as you go along and using a set order of discussion for handover will help to avoid errors and omissions. The role of electronic referral systems in the documentation of both the referral and the response is widely valued in the organisation of these complex tasks.

References

1. General Medical Council. Domain 3 – Colleagues, Culture and Safety: Good Medical Practice (Domain 3 Colleagues Culture and Safety – GMC). gmc-uk.org. Accessed 7 June 2024.

2. Black Country Partnership. Clinical Handover. www.bcpft.nhs.uk/documents/policies/h/1386-handover-clinical/file#:~:text=Clinical%20Handover%20%2D%20A%20semi%2Dstructured,take%20place%20in%20different%20ways. Accessed 27 November 2023.

3. Royal College of Surgeons of England. Safe Handover: Guidance from the Working Time Direcrtive Working Party. https://www.rcseng.ac.uk/library-and-publications/rcs-publications/docs/safe-handover/#:~:text=The%20transfer%20of%20a%20patient,the%20duty%20of%20every%20doctor. Published March 2007.

4. CQC Compliance. Clinical Governance. https://cqc-compliance.com/clinical-governance/. Accessed 27 November 2023.

5. Australian Nursing & Midwifery Journal. 5 Tips to a Good Clinical Handover. https://anmj.org.au/5-tips-to-a-good-clinical-handover/. Accessed 27 November 2023.

6. R. Bradley, M. Bremner, A. McKindley and S. Lammy. Usefulness of Royal College of Surgeons of England Operation Note Guidelines to Neurosurgical Practice: A Closed Loop Audit. Br J Neurosurg. 2021; 35(4):418–423.

Acknowledgements

We wish to express our thanks to Cambridge University Press and to thank our colleagues in Glasgow for their continued and ongoing support to ensure the handover of neurosurgical patients at the Institute of Neurological Sciences remains of a consistently high level.

Cambridge Elements ≡

Emergency Neurosurgery

Nihal Gurusinghe

Lancashire Teaching Hospital NHS Trust

Professor Nihal Gurusinghe is a Consultant Neurosurgeon at the Lancashire Teaching Hospitals NHS Trust. He is on the Executive Council of the Society of British Neurological Surgeons as the Lead for NICE (National Institute for Health and Care Excellence) guidelines relating to neurosurgical practice. He is also an examiner for the UK and International FRCS examinations in Neurosurgery.

Peter Hutchinson

University of Cambridge, Society of British Neurological Surgeons and Royal College of Surgeons of England

Peter Hutchinson BSc MBBS FFSEM FRCS(SN) PhD FMedSci is Professor of Neurosurgery and Head of the Division of Academic Neurosurgery at the University of Cambridge, and Honorary Consultant Neurosurgeon at Addenbrooke's Hospital. He is Director of Clinical Research at the Royal College of Surgeons of England and Meetings Secretary of the Society of British Neurological Surgeons.

Ioannis Fouyas

Royal College of Surgeons of Edinburgh

Ioannis Fouyas is a Consultant Neurosurgeon in Edinburgh. His clinical interests focus on the treatment of complex cerebrovascular and skull base pathologies. His academic endeavours concentrate in the field of cerebrovascular pathophysiology. His passion is technical surgical training, fulfilled in collaboration with the Royal College of Surgeons of Edinburgh. Finally, he pursues Undergraduate Neuroscience teaching, with a particular focus on functional Neuroanatomy.

Naomi Slator

North Bristol NHS Trust

Naomi Slator FRCS (SN) is a Consultant Spinal Neurosurgeon based at North Bristol NHS Trust. She has a specialist interest in Complex Spine alongside Cranial and Spinal Trauma. She completed her neurosurgical training in Birmingham and a six-month Fellowship in CSF and Trauma (2019). She then went on to complete her Spinal Fellowship in Leeds (2020) before moving to the southwest to take up her consultant post.

Ian Kamaly-Asl

Royal Manchester Children's Hospital

Ian Kamaly-Asl is a full time paediatric neurosurgeon and Honorary Chair at Royal Manchester Children's Hospital. He trained in North Western Deanery with fellowships at Boston Children's Hospital and Sick Kids in Toronto. Ian is a member of council of The Royal College of Surgeons of England and The SBNS where he is lead for mentoring and tackling oppressive behaviours.

Peter Whitfield

University Hospitals Plymouth NHS Trust

Professor Peter Whitfield is a Consultant Neurosurgeon at the South West Neurosurgical Centre, University Hospitals Plymouth NHS Trust. His clinical interests include vascular neurosurgery, neuro oncology and trauma. He has held many roles in postgraduate neurosurgical education and is President of the Society of British Neurological Surgeons. Peter has published widely, and is passionate about education, training and the promotion of clinical research.

About the Series

Elements in Emergency Neurosurgery is intended for trainees and practitioners in Neurosurgery and Emergency Medicine as well as allied specialties all over the world. Authored by international experts, this series provides core knowledge, common clinical pathways and recommendations on the management of acute conditions of the brain and spine.

Cambridge Elements ≡

Emergency Neurosurgery

Elements in the Series

A full series listing is available at: www.cambridge.org/EEMN

Printed in the United States
by Baker & Taylor Publisher Services